The Rt Hon David Ennals MP,

Secretary of State for Social Services

1. We submit the attached proposals in accordance with the obligations placed upon us by Section 68 of the National Health Service Act 1977.

2. These proposals are based on evidence of the existence of suitable alternative accommodation outside the NHS hospitals under consideration to accommodate at least a part of the demand for private medicine currently directed towards the pay beds in those hospitals. Before making these proposals we obtained information on the facilities, and the extent of spare capacity, available at a number of private hospitals throughout the country. We then considered which private hospitals could reasonably be expected to serve as suitable alternatives to a specific number of pay beds in particular NHS hospitals. The information available to us for this purpose was sufficient for us to issue successive groups of provisional proposals to a number of health authorities and other interested parties in England, and to seek their comments on them. A period of three months was allowed for representations to be made to us in respect of each provisional proposal. We then reconsidered a number of our first group of provisional proposals in the light of all the evidence we received. The proposals now submitted, therefore, represent only the first instalment of those based on spare capacity in private hospitals. We intend to submit further proposals at three monthly intervals.

3. In many instances representations were made to us that some of the patients currently being treated in pay beds were suffering from conditions, which could not be treated in the private hospital proposed as an alternative, or that their treatment needed equipment or other facilities which the private hospital lacked. On a number of occasions the objectors specifically referred to cases which would be covered by Section 59 of the 1977 Act once the Government have put it into operation. Their delay in doing this is giving rise to certain misconceptions. For example, many people think that pay beds need to be retained for patients who are to be admitted under Section 59, whereas there is no requirement that patients admitted under that Section have to be admitted to authorised pay beds. There is also a danger that people may have expectations that Section 59 admission arrangements will cover a far wider range of patients than will prove to be the case.

4. In the introduction to our second set of proposals, submitted to you on 29 March 1978, we urged the early and widespread introduction of admission arrangements under Section 59. We can only repeat this request and remind you that, until this is done, we may find ourselves obliged to retain more pay beds than the operation of Section 59 will eventually show to be justified.

5. You will see that we propose implementation of our revocation proposals before 1 July 1979. Although we do not have statutory power to propose a date on which the proposals should be implemented, we recommend that these proposals should not be implemented before 30 June 1979.

6. We should be grateful if you would publish this covering note with our detailed proposals.

<table>
<tr><td>WIGODER</td><td>CYRIL SCURR</td></tr>
<tr><td>RAY BUCKTON</td><td>DEREK STEVENSON</td></tr>
<tr><td>BERNARD DIX</td><td></td></tr>
</table>

26 March 1979.

HEALTH SERVICES BOARD PROPOSALS
MARCH 1979—ENGLAND
PRIVATE RESIDENT PATIENTS

The Health Services Board propose that authorisations granted under Section 65(1) of the National Health Service Act 1977, for the use of accommodation at NHS hospitals for private resident patients, at hospitals or groups of hospitals in England shall be revoked before 1 July 1979 in the manner and to the extent specified in the entries on this page and the following page respectively.

SOUTH EAST THAMES REGIONAL HEALTH AUTHORITY

1. *East Sussex Area Health Authority*

The group authorisation for Hastings Health District shall be revoked to the extent of reducing the number of authorised beds from 9 to 6 and the authorisations for Royal East Sussex Hospital, Buchanan Hospital, Bexhill Hospital and Rye, Winchelsea and District Memorial Hospital shall be revoked to the extent of reducing the number of authorised beds from 8 to 6, from 4 to 2, from 3 to NIL and from 1 to NIL respectively.

2. *Kent Area Health Authority*

The group authorisation for South East Kent Health District shall be revoked to the extent of reducing the number of authorised beds from 10 to 3 and the authorisation for Ashford Hospital shall be revoked to the extent of reducing the number of authorised beds from 6 to 3.

SOUTH WESTERN REGIONAL HEALTH AUTHORITY

3. *Gloucestershire Area Health Authority*

The group authorisation for Gloucestershire Area shall be revoked to the extent of reducing the number of authorised beds from 32 to 23.

WEST MIDLANDS REGIONAL HEALTH AUTHORITY

4. *Salop Area Health Authority*

The group authorisation for Salop Area shall be revoked to the extent of reducing the number of authorised beds from 5 to 4 and the authorisation for the Royal Shrewsbury Hospital Copthorne (South) shall be revoked to the extent of reducing the number of authorised beds from 5 to 4.

5. *Staffordshire Area Health Authority*

The group authorisation for North Staffordshire Health District shall be revoked to the extent of reducing the number of authorised beds from 22 to 10 and the group authorisation for North Staffordshire Royal Infirmary, Hartshill Orthopaedic Hospital and the City General Hospital shall be revoked to the extent of reducing the number of authorised beds from 22 to 10.

6. *Wolverhampton Area Health Authority*

The group authorisation for Wolverhampton Area shall be revoked to the extent of reducing the number of authorised beds from 21 to 7 and the authorisations for Queen Victoria Nursing Institution and New Cross Hospital shall be revoked to the extent of reducing the number of authorised beds from 21 to 3 and from 5 to 3 respectively.

MERSEY REGIONAL HEALTH AUTHORITY

7. *Cheshire Area Health Authority*

The group authorisation for Chester Health District shall be revoked to the extent of reducing the number of authorised beds from 5 to 2 and the authorisations for West Cheshire Hospital (Maternity) and Chester Royal Infirmary shall be revoked to the extent of reducing the number of authorised beds from 4 to 1 and from 5 to 2 respectively.

The effect of these proposals is to reduce by 49 the number of authorised beds which may be occupied at any one time in England.

Printed in England for Her Majesty's Stationery Office by Oyez Press Limited
Dd. 294608 · K32 6/79

HER MAJESTY'S STATIONERY OFFICE

Government Bookshops

49 High Holborn, London WC1V 6HB
13a Castle Street, Edinburgh EH2 3AR
41 The Hayes, Cardiff CF1 1JW
Brazennose Street, Manchester M60 8AS
Southey House, Wine Street, Bristol BS1 2BQ
258 Broad Street, Birmingham B1 2HE
80 Chichester Street, Belfast BT1 4JY

*Government publications are also available
through booksellers*

Withdrawal of Authorisations for the use of NHS Hospital Accommodation and Services by Private Patients-Health Services Board's Fifth Set of Proposals

PROPOSALS MADE BY THE HEALTH SERVICES BOARD UNDER SECTION 68 OF THE NATIONAL HEALTH SERVICE ACT 1977 (c. 49) IN RESPECT OF ENGLAND

Presented to Parliament pursuant to Section 74 of the National Health Service Act 1977, by the Secretary of State for Social Services

---

Ordered by The House of Commons *to be printed*
25th May 1979

LONDON
HER MAJESTY'S STATIONERY OFFICE
25p net

H.C. 17

ISBN 0 10 201780 8